Clients and Their Caregivers

Helpful Tips from a "Quadriplegic"

by

Kawand S. Crawford

To contact author:

donkawand@aol.com

facebook.com/authorkawand

www.donkawand.com

twitter.com/Donkawand

Donkawand Publications, LLC

Acknowledgments

I would like to thank God for giving me the strength and support needed to live life as independent as possible.

Clients and Their Caregivers
Helpful Tips from a "Quadriplegic"

by Kawand S Crawford

Chapter 1

Minor Adjustments

My name is Kawand S. Crawford and at this point in my life I've been paralyzed for over 20 years. I was diagnosed as a quadriplegic, someone who lacks feelings and mobility from the chest down, which makes me very dependent on a Caregiver. Some people might refer to them as home health aides, home attendant or CNA (certified nurse's assistant).

The word is kind of broad and really could include babysitters or anyone providing some form of care to another individual. I have worked with people with different credentials so I think it's always a good idea to ask for their credentials and what they prefer to be called.

For the purpose of simplicity, I will refer to individuals who care for people with disabilities as Caregiver's. I will also refer to the individuals with disabilities that receive some kind of personal health services as the Client. I believe a Caregiver and Client have a very unique relationship especially in a home setting.

A Caregiver is someone who cares for people with specific medical needs in either a Hospital setting or within a private home. Many have told me that they prefer and enjoy working in a home setting. They like the one-on-one care as opposed to the Hospital where they may be responsible for many different patients or Clients.

As a person with a physical disability and Client, I also prefer the home setting. Shortly after being paralyzed, I spent over a year and a half at Goldwater Memorial Hospital, a Rehabilitation Center in NYC. At one point I was in a ward that housed close to 80 patients. There were about three or four nurses on staff at any given moment. It's a situation that affected the level of care individuals with disabilities needed.

Since becoming paralyzed, I've lived in two different states, worked with at least a half a dozen different healthcare agencies and plenty of different Caregiver's. I've dealt with many different ethnic groups and personalities. And just like any other profession, you will find some very bad ones.

I've had the pleasure of working with some extraordinary people. I've also some very good relationships with most of them. Unfortunately I ran cross some shady ones and then I've worked with some downright foolish ones.

I believe that if a person lives long enough, they will either know someone that needs some kind of personal assistance with their daily activities or need one of them self. It's unfortunate, but it's reality. We take our God-given abilities for granted until it hits home. When it does hit home it opens up a whole other world.

I've had friends tell me that after I became paralyzed they became more conscious of people with disabilities around them. Every day there is someone whose life changes drastically by illness, accident or victim of a crime. It's a life altering experience that no one is totally prepared for.

I found that most people have someone in their family that relies on a Caregiver. Therefore there are several very important tips that I would like to share if you ever have to depend on a Caregiver or knows someone who does. These tips are beneficial to both

Caregivers and those who need them.

Keep in mind as you read some of my personal experiences that everyone's situation is different, although I do believe that there are some fundamental things that can help provide a long-lasting work relationship between a Client and a Caregiver.

Let me start by telling you a little bit about a Caregiver. A Caregiver is usually someone with a little medical knowledge that likes to assist people with disabilities with their daily activities. They usually prefer to work in someone's home as opposed to working in a nursing home. They are generally employed by a healthcare agency and basically work as Independent Contractors (depending on the company).

Outside of some mandatory weekends and/or holidays, they pretty much work when they want. They pick the time and days that they are available to work and they pick which Clients they would like to continue working for after the first day. This is something that I believe contributes to some discrimination. As a person in the healthcare field you're going to have to work with people with different paralysis. I found that the more assistance a Client needs the less a Caregiver wants to work for them. It's a problem I've run into several times.

A Caregiver has the right to not want to continue working with a particular Client and they will be moved to another Client. There are some situations that might really warrant a Caregiver to not want to continue working with the Client in their home. The first is IF and only IF the Caregiver believes that their life or well-being is being compromised. The second one is if a Client or their family members are verbally abusive towards the Caregiver.

Whenever a Caregiver doesn't want to remain on the case, it is a change that has to go through a Coordinator at the healthcare agency. Now, I'm sure that not working for particular Clients with certain paralysis is not what a Caregiver tells the Coordinator. Someone might beg to differ, but I've had plenty of people in the field mention to me that a lot of Caregiver's do not like working with quadriplegics or someone with a disability that requires a great deal of assistance.

When a Caregiver has too many legitimate complaints or grievances against a Client there is usually what I call a "Powwow Meeting". It's a meeting between the agencies Director, Coordinator, Client and Case Manager. A close family member or spouse could also sit in on this meeting.

As a Client living in Georgia, I am on a program called ICWP (Independent Care Waiver

Program) which provides me with a case manager that acts as a liaison between the healthcare agency and me. They perform some of the same functions as a Social worker. Both the Caregiver's and Clients' grievances are usually addressed at the "Powwow" meeting.

This is a meeting that I've been involved with myself a couple of times during my early years of being paralyzed. I really didn't understand how the system worked and thought that although I was paralyzed I could still be the person that I used to be. This is something that is really not true.

Yes, I learned early that a Caregiver has a responsibility to report what goes on in a Client's home to their coordinator. Most of this information is kept on record and usually comes up at one of these meetings.

For example, when I was in my early 20's, I enjoyed listening to some hard-core rap music.

Sometimes I'd like to listen to songs with some very strong language and, I must admit, a little disrespectful to women. It's just the kind of music that I preferred. It's also something that could make a Caregiver a little uncomfortable and eventually drop you as a Client.

It took some time to understand that if I wanted to maintain a long-lasting working relationship with a Caregiver that I would sometimes have to make some minor adjustments in my life. So today I am conscious of the kind of music I play around my Caregivers. I usually try to find out what genre of music they like our initial meeting just to nip that situation in the bud.

I was a young thug from the streets, so being snitched (reported) on truly frustrated me. It seems petty but if I wanted longevity with a caregiver I had to be mindful of the music I played.

It helps to be versatile. Therefore, my music choices span cross different genres. But if you're a young or older person who likes what you like this can become a problem. Now, I'm sure many may say, "It's my house... I pay rent and I can listen to what I like" which may be true, but remember, your home is now someone's workplace.

There must be some kind type of compromise when it comes to something so personal to both people. If you've ever had a job before you know that every workplace has policies in place to help create a balanced working environment for everyone.

Now, they may tell you they don't mind what you're listening to but I found that not to be true in some cases. Remember that it's their job and they might tell you what they think you want to hear to keep it. You have to constantly keep in mind that although it is your house, it is also their workplace.

I found that when I meet a Caregiver that enjoys the same kind of music I do we usually have a much better relationship than someone who doesn't. I used music as an example because it also helps to create a more relaxed and motivating environment.

For example, before I was paralyzed and like most young people I enjoyed listening to music whenever I cleaned up around the house. The music not only motivated me but also made the time go by much quicker. I've noticed that the same is true when I have a Caregiver that likes my kind of music. Their performance is more efficient and their attitude is usually positive. Working with someone with a positive attitude always creates a healthy and happy environment.

Music is also good for the soul because not only can it motivate you but it can also comfort you during some tough moments.

Whether it's the Client or Caregiver having a bad day a little soft music usually brings a person back down-to-earth.

One of the things that keep me comfortable as a quadriplegic is stability. It's one of the most important things for a person with a disability and their family.

As a Client you can listen to the music you like when you're Caregiver is not around. It's a minor adjustment that's really temporary until a Client meets someone who enjoys the music they do.

If listening to the kind of music you like is truly important you can always invest in some headphones. Sometimes we have to make changes in ourselves in order to improve our quality of life. Having a disability already diminishes your quality of life so it helps to incorporate anything in your day to make living with a disability just a little more comfortable.

Making a minor adjustment such as when and what kind of music to play in front of a Caregiver can take the interaction a long way. It's a small price for a quadriplegic or someone with a disability to pay to keep someone around.

Chapter 2

Not a Maid

Most of the Caregiver's that I have encountered have a real and legitimate problem when you refer to them as a maid. Referring to them as a maid is extremely insulting just as if someone called me a cripple. Unfortunately, we live in a time where most people would like for you to be politically correct. Therefore Clients, family and friends should not refer to them as a maid. This is an assumption that most folks that are not familiar with the profession usually think.

A Client can also have this misconception when their spinal cord injury or disability is brand-new. It's not the Client's intent but the lack of knowledge. Unless you were actually born with a disability, going from being able and independent to disabled, changes your everyday life as you once knew it. It's definitely a new way of living. No matter how intelligent you are you have to learn to live all over again. Understanding the role of a Caregiver is something that has to be learned.

Yes, some light cleaning is part of their job description (depending on the Client) but it doesn't make them a maid. I've heard plenty of stories about Clients that might have had a stroke or some other kind of severe paralysis where they are pretty independent and only need assistance with some light cleaning. What most Clients, friends and family don't understand is that although this individual is doing some light cleaning for a particular Client it is for that Client **"ONLY!"**

A Client should understand that they are the ones receiving the service that's being provided because of a particular disability. Caregivers go out to a person's home to assist with whatever the Client is unable to do for them self. They are not responsible or obligated to assist individuals that are able-bodied. This could become a serious problem for a Caregiver, especially when working in someone's home that is shared by other people, which is the case most of the time.

I must confess that when I became paralyzed I thought of a Caregiver as a person who had an obligation to keep my house clean. In my mind I believed it meant cleaning up behind all my friends but I was wrong! Having friends over is a beautiful thing but a Client, their friends and family should "not" expect them to clean behind "groups" of people.

When I first began receiving assistance I was young and extremely popular. I had a great deal of people I considered friends stopping by to visit on a daily basis. At the time I was unaware that most Caregiver's like the job because of the one-on-one care they provide to a particular individual. The key word is "individual" and both my friends and I took this part of the job for granted. I don't believe it was something we did on purpose but didn't fully understand since no one had ever been around a Caregiver before.

I remember debating with the Director of a healthcare agency during a Powwow meeting that I could not control how my friends left my apartment after visiting, but that was not true. I was young, immature and enjoyed having groups of people at my home just hanging out. I had my own apartment so my place had become the hangout spot.

I put my friends before my quality of life, instead of the other way around. A part of me was concerned that my friends wouldn't come around if I asked them to clean up after themselves whenever they visited. The truth is I found out who my real friends were. I had to realize that I wasn't asking them to clean up my house but their own mess, something that is taught to most of us as children.

As a Client, you have to ask those that visit to respect your place. It is only courteous and responsible for any adult/child visiting another person. This is a conversation that a Client should have with those they consider to be friends. They have to understand that the Caregiver is there to help with the Clients quality of life.

Sometimes the people around us that we call friends don't have our best interests at heart. Most people just don't know exactly what a Caregiver's responsibilities are. A

Client may be concerned about folks not visiting, but real friends will understand and those that don't are not really friends and shouldn't be welcomed. It really comes down to just basic home training, something I found a lot of people don't have. Asking folks to respect the cleanliness of your place might cost you a few people but can open your eyes to true friendship.

It will also enhance your quality of life. Your furniture and personal things last longer and your place stays cleaner. Being clean is a necessity for a quadriplegic. Since a quadriplegic is unable to move, it can get real interesting if the home is infested with cockroaches. I know for me it's difficult to go to sleep after I spotted one anywhere that I have to sleep. Hate to have one crawling on me and I can't swipe it away. The previous scenario is something that most people without a spinal cord injury take for granted.

Today I have a small group of quality friends that stuck by my side for over 20 years and truly understand and respect my new way of living. It takes a special person to be a friend to someone with a spinal cord injury. This friend has to respect and understand that Caregivers are there for the Client only.

I have not met a Caregiver who will break this one particular rule of cleaning up behind anyone other than the Client. Most have told me that they might clean up behind friends or family members as a favor once in a while. It's not something they do often out of fear that once they do it, it would become something to be expected. Therefore, most of them "never" clean up after friends or family members.

A Client may sacrifice a long-lasting relationship with a good

Caregiver if they do not have this talk with those that are closest to them. It is something that a Client really should consider before they find themselves living in a filthy home or, even worse, unable to receive any assistance. Not being able to receive services is the worst-case scenario but sincerely realistic.

Now if you're a filthy Client who really doesn't care about how you're living then eventually it will be difficult for you to maintain a long-lasting relationship with any Caregiver. Don't get me wrong, one might hang around for a couple of weeks but eventually the Client will have to start all over. Not unless the Client gets a Caregiver who is just as filthy as the Client.

I usually mention to all of my new Caregivers on the first day that I'm no neat freak, but I'm no slob. I believe the majority of people fit the previous category. There are your neat fanatics that are probably suffering from Obsessive Compulsive Disorder (OCD) just like there are individuals that hoard everything. It would help to be someone that lives in the middle but each Client has their own quality of life that they prefer living.

Unfortunately who we were before spinal cord injuries or any other disability is who we are afterwards when it comes to being a clean person. Our cleaning habits are adapted over time and as people I believe we get stuck and what's normal for us. The majority of the Caregiver's I've encountered prefer a clean and orderly place to work.

Therefore, designating days throughout the week to help maintain a clean home would be a good idea. The amount of days needed could vary depending on how much company a Client has. The previous scenario only works for a Client who lives by their self. A Caregiver will and I mean religiously only keep clean the area they use or the Client occupies. I do believe that there should be an exception to the rule.

I think that there is a difference between having friends and family over every day and someone who stops by periodically. Of course having people in and out of your home all day every day will contribute to the dysfunction of your place and a Caregiver should not be responsible.

Let's say someone stops by every so often for a few minutes and asked for a glass of water. A quadriplegic is unable to assist so their guest either has to go in the kitchen themselves or rely on their Caregiver. After drinking the water a Client and their guest are engaged in a conversation that last a couple of minutes before they get up and leave. They are joking and laughing on their way out and unconsciously leave behind the glass.

I found that most Caregivers do not mind cleaning behind someone in the previous example, but there are some that will leave that glass right where it is. It may sound crazy but something I have experienced many times before. As long as I've been receiving assistance, most people who have visited me will leave something behind. Most of the Caregiver's I've had more than one day will also eventually leave something behind. It's something that just happens.

I've also known for a Caregiver not to clean up behind others Caregiver's who might have left something. It confuses me because they work for the same company and the cleanliness of a Clients place reflects on the quality of services provided by their agency.

A Client may find them self in a position where more than one Caregiver will enter the home. It can be within the same day or one may come for a couple of days and another on other days. Working with more than one Caregiver in a particular day can get a little frustrating. I also found it to be an on-going issue because there is always something that needs cleaning in a home where people live. I get the impression that they expect a Client's place to be exactly the way they left it, which is impossible. Cleaning up behind other folks is an issue that had been brought to my attention in a Powwow meeting several times during my first few years of being paralyzed.

One day a meeting was taking place in my bedroom on a day that I preferred not to get up. Therefore the Director, Coordinator and my Case Manager had to bring chairs from my dining room table into my bedroom. After discussing all of the issues they all got up and left my room. I waited patiently until they got near my front door before calling the Director of the health care agency back.

When the middle-age lady returned to my bedroom, I politely asked her, "Now who is supposed to remove these chairs?" She got a good laugh out of it, although I was serious. Sometimes in life it's easier to show someone what you're talking about than telling them. I believe I made my point, which is that sometimes when someone is not used to visiting you how easy it is to leave something behind in the midst of saying goodbye.

Like I said earlier, this is a situation in which someone that doesn't normally stop by does. Since I am a quadriplegic, when the Director inadvertently left her chair, someone had to be responsible for moving it. This is a scenario that I discuss with most of my Caregivers just in case it occurs. It is a judgment call by a Caregiver that most do not have a problem with. The cleanup is usually minor but still needed for someone *living with a* physical disability.

As a quadriplegic, my Caregivers are more to me than just someone who cleans my house. Working with an individual *who has a severe* physical disability may require assistance with *their* personal hygiene, running errands, cooking and at times, emotional support. If you're lucky to have a Caregiver longer than 90 days, they will probably be around you when you're experiencing some form of depression. If they talk you through what you're going through it doesn't make them a psychologist and because they help to prepare meals doesn't make them a chef.

If a Client addresses this issue with his family and friends early it can help make for a longer working relationship between a Client and Caregiver. *A* Caregiver should use common sense when it comes to having to clean up behind a guest. Most understand the difference between a guest that rarely stops by and a group of people who show up daily and abuse the Client's personal space.

Having a clean home creates an environment that most Caregivers are comfortable working in. Remember when they're entering your home for the first time it's the first thing they notice. It's at that point they began to assess how long they would like to work with a *Client*.

Chapter 3

Money or Love

Although I've dealt with hundreds of Caregiver's I can pretty much and safely say that I can put them into two categories. There are those that do it for the money and those who do it for the love. The group of people who are in it for the money don't mind going through the brief training classes in order to get work. It is not a profession that requires a great deal of education if any at all which is why I believe it contributes to a few bad apples slipping through.

The ones that enter into this profession just for the money really do a disservice to the company that they work for and the Client. It is something that could affect their work performance. One of the things that I noticed in this type of individual is their unwillingness to work.

One good sign is that they will wait to be instructed on each and every specific task. They rarely initiate anything that might provide some work for them. You might not notice the first day or two because they are motivated by the money. But it won't be long before you begin to notice that they will enter your apartment and wait for you to ask and be specific on what it is that you need.

Less say that the Client is on the phone when they first come in and having a really deep conversation. Caregivers that are in it for the money will have a seat and wait for the Client to finish. Now on the surface it seems like there's really nothing wrong with this when a Caregiver enters a *Client*'s house because you might not know what a Client needs or would like you to do. This is something a Client can expect from an individual within the first week or two. But if a Caregiver has worked with a Client for at least two weeks there are some basic things that *they* can initiate without being asked.

For example as a quadriplegic I rely on a Caregiver to assist with bathing. Normally I take a basic bed bath and I have particular days throughout the week when I take showers. I usually let my Caregiver know the day before if I plan to take a shower. Very seldom, although it has happened will I spring it on them on that particular day. I do this because I like to give them the opportunity to bring the proper footwear because given a quadriplegic a shower can get messy from the knees down.

Now I've had Caregiver's tell me that they have had Clients that don't like to bathe on a daily basis which is an ideal Client for someone who's in it for the money but that is not most cases. As much as I dread having to depend on someone to provide this service for me it is something that I do not skip.

If a Caregiver enters the home of a quadriplegic in the morning or someone who needs assistance with bathing, preparing for this activity is routine. It's a task that a Client should not have to ask a Caregiver to perform. If they've been in a Client's home for at least a week they already know where everything is located.

Most Clients keep their cosmetics in the bathroom like a normal person and their medical supplies close by. So while the Client is on the phone the Caregiver could be getting everything together but instead will sit and wait for the Client to finish before preparing to assist with bathing.

Now some might argue that maybe the Client is not ready to wash up immediately after getting off the phone but the reality is no matter when, bathing is something that a Client needs daily. Therefore not knowing if or when a Client wants to bathe immediately after getting off the phone is just a poor excuse and a good sign of a person that's in the business for the money.

I'm not going to sit here and tell you that everyone who is in the business for the money does this but most of the individuals that I have encountered with this habit usually got the job just for the paycheck. It is also a very good sign of a lazy person. If you're lazy you should avoid this profession and especially a Client such as a quadriplegic who needs "constant" assistance. Working for a quadriplegic or anyone who depends on you to help with their quality of life is demanding.

The same goes for cleaning around the apartment. A Client shouldn't have to ask you to sweep the floors if and when there dirty. Once a Client has established with a Caregiver that they are not a slob it should be automatic, something a

Caregiver should know about a Client in the first week. That's just my opinion! Cleaning is a task that can be done at any given time and especially if the Client is on the phone or engaged in some other activity during your first few minutes in their home.

I've also notice that they pay very close attention to the time they get off. They will leave on time each and every day or you will begin to see some attitude. If this happens it won't be long before they drop the Client. Some will even try to leave before their scheduled time. Now don't get me wrong if you do not get paid for overtime you should be ready and able to leave when you've completed your time.

Unfortunately being a Caregiver in a home setting might require you to leave late sometimes. You may be involved in a task just before your time to leave that needs you to stay later. As a quadriplegic there are many things that can go wrong with me just before your shift is over. It's just something that's a part of the job and the life of a quadriplegic.

I have heard plenty of Caregiver's who believe that some Clients make a habit of it. Some Clients can take a Caregiver's time to leave for granted something else that I'm guilty of doing during my first several years. I wasn't doing it on purpose I just didn't realize or give it any thought that the Caregiver's have a life after they leave.

All Clients should allow themselves at least 30 min. before the end of the shift to begin preparing for their exit. I think 30 min. is enough time for you to take any necessary medications, have a snack and made comfortable. This is something that I have learned to do over the years and recommend that most Clients adopt in order to create a healthier relationship. And just like a Client prefers for them to be on time they also like to leave on time.

Finally a person who's just in it for the check, work performance is usually half ass. This is something that would be obvious to you, your family and other Caregiver's if you have more than one within the same day. If you're not a person who loves taking care of people please find another profession because you are responsible for the quality of life for another individual. It's almost the same as having a baby and still wanting to be in the clubs "every" night. Not good!

The second category of Caregiver's and the ones that seem to last the longest absolutely love taking care of people. I found that I've had a much better and long-lasting relationship with this group because although they probably could use the paycheck they love what they do. This has to be a person with a great deal of patience and compassion.

This kind of individual feels right at home after about a week. They initiate dialogue pertaining to a Client's care and daily activities. If this individual entered a Client's home after working for about a week and the Client is on the phone, would automatically begin to do things to prepare themselves for the Client's daily activities. The more they get to know a Client's routine the more they began to initiate the basic tasks. This is a person who after a few minutes of not doing anything would ask, "Are you okay and do you need me to do anything?"

The really good just to ask the previous question constantly which is something that I like. Sometimes I'm not in the mood to be asking for help. As a quadriplegic I am constantly asking for assistance and sometimes I just don't feel like asking. I'm sure that I'm not the only Client who feels like this sometimes. Before I became paralyzed I was independent and always had trouble asking people for help. Therefore, I found that I get more done working with someone who initiates activities on their own. It gives me a break from having to ask for the things I need.

This type of Caregiver will not have a problem with staying a few minutes after their time. Most of them will not leave until a Client is absolutely comfortable. And to be honest sometimes you may have to politely put them out.

It usually takes a medical emergency or having to pick up their children when they get off that time becomes an issue. If a Caregiver has to leave on time it's something that they notify the Client of in advance. They will also let a Client know what days they will not be working.

This is something that I personally appreciate because I'm

able to prepare myself mentally for a stranger to enter my home. They are not obligated to let a Client know but understand the importance of stability. They also care about who's coming to work in their place. Unlike someone who just takes the day off and doesn't mention it to their Client. (Here is another good sign of a Caregiver who's in it for the money.)

All of the good Caregiver's are hospitable to everyone that enters a Clients home. Probably because they love people in general or know that when you give blessings to others you receive them. Whatever it is, they are sociable with people which make a quadriplegic or someone with a severe disability life more livable. It also makes the people visiting their loved ones just a little more comfortable about the care their loved ones are receiving.

Finally, a Client is usually satisfied with their work performance, everything from their level of care when bathing to maintaining a respectable place. The good Caregiver's can have a bad day and still perform professionally. Everyone has a moment that's outside of their character but it doesn't last long when you're a positive thinking person.

A good friend of mines and a quadriplegic himself up until his passing a couple years ago told me, "A person's character will not allow them to be other than they are." - Luis Rodriguez

If you're someone who loves people no matter how frustrated you get in your personal life or on the job your character will not allow you to mistreat a Client. I believe after about a week of being around someone you can tell if there in it for the money or the love. When I meet one who loves what they do, it improves my quality of life.

Chapter 4

Family and Friends

I am a child of God and I have been blessed throughout my life with an extraordinary family and good friends. Being a quadriplegic is rough emotionally and every day is challenging. Having a Caregiver helps me to be independent but also allows my family and friends to not worry about me while they're living their own lives. I know that I'm blessed because my family and friends have displayed a great deal of support since I've been paralyzed.

When someone has a physical or mental disability it's important for family and friends to be around. Even though there are some very good Caregiver's as a Client you must always keep in mind that it's just a job for them. They need time off, have personal issues at home which might force them to be late or have to leave early. So when a Client can't count on the Caregiver, their family and friends are very important. They should assist with their loved ones personal things outside of a Caregiver's job description.

A Client may have some personal hobbies or be a person who likes pets. No matter how much a Caregiver may love their job, there are some things they may feel uncomfortable doing. If you find that there are some personal activities that a Caregiver is uncomfortable with as a Client the less you have them do this activity the longer they will last. A person is not going to do something that they hate to do but for so long. Therefore if they make a comment or display an expression of disgust a Client might want to consider getting assistance from a family member or friend.

For example I was going through a phase for about 10 years when I was in love with having a large aquarium in my apartment. Helping to maintain my aquarium was considered something out of a Caregiver's job description. I've been blessed to have some Caregiver's that would help from time to time but I always asked someone in the family or a friend to help in between.

I believe when the health care agency or those individuals who founded the system and wrote their policies didn't consider a hobby a necessity. I guess the idea was that a person with a disability should be happy just receiving assistance with their personal care. Everyone has hobbies or things outside of their personal care that they like or love.

Every little thing that interests a Client contributes to their emotional stability. For me watching my fish swim or just hearing the filter run softly at night was very therapeutic. It might not seem like much to a Caregiver or Health Care Agency but the more stable a Client is emotionally the easier they are to deal with. Everybody has something that they like that other people might not understand but makes them feel good even if it's for a moment.

Good friends and family are just like good Caregiver's. They engage me and initiate activities. They call and check on me constantly instead of waiting for me to call and ask for something I may need. They invite me to go places and even if I'm with a Caregiver don't mind helping to care for me. When a Caregiver sees that they have a Client whose family and friends generally care for them it makes them care just a little bit more.

As a quadriplegic it's good to have quality friends and supportive family. Let's say for example a Caregiver is on their way to work and their child has an asthma attack and has to be rushed to the hospital. When they contact the coordinator at the health care agency it can take a few hours before someone else shows up.

A Client should have someone they can call in case of an emergency. Even if it's only to make them comfortable and keep them emotionally stable. Most Caregiver's are women that have kids so there's always a chance of an emergency coming up. A Caregiver not showing up or running a little late on a very important day could be tragic. I know that there are Clients and family members who expect the Caregiver's to do everything but those expectations are not realistic.

In order to keep a Caregiver around for a little while you should learn quickly what it is that they don't like doing and feel strongly about. Let's say a Client lives in an apartment that has an attic. A good

Caregiver might not like going up the flimsy staircase that leads to the attic, a legitimate fear but not enough for a Client to replace her/him. A Client can put whatever they want in the attic in a corner until a family member or friend has time.

A Client should not be angry or bent out of shape with what makes a Caregiver uncomfortable because as people we all have our limitations whether it's because where afraid or just don't feel comfortable. A Client along with friends and family must respect and be a little more understanding to what a Caregiver is not required to do or uncomfortable with doing. That's what a friend or family is for.

Family members and friends in my opinion can recognize when a loved one is being cared for properly. Both family and friends should not mind contributing to improving the quality of life for their loved ones. Unfortunately not everyone has family support or good friends and therefore must rely on their Caregiver even more.

The previous scenario makes a person with a disability vulnerable for abuse. The less family and friends come around the more control a Caregiver has over a Client, depending on the Client's mental abilities. It may sound unthinkable but unfortunately some people will take advantage of someone with a disability. It is something that I witnessed during my long stay in the hospital after having my accident. I've also seen plenty of specials on television shows like 20/20 where they set up hidden cameras and catch the abuse on camera. And shame on them!

As a quadriplegic I am vulnerable to those that don't have my well-being in heart. Some Caregiver's can be intimidating and somewhat controlling. Just the presence of your family and friends can prevent some abuse. Living life with a disability is something that requires assistance outside of the Caregiver's. This is where the people who love someone with a disability should step in to the picture.

Chapter 5

First Meeting

I remember the anxiety of meeting my first Caregiver ever like it was yesterday. And believe it or not after 20 years I still feel some anxiety when meeting someone new. I was in my early 20s and still had the smell of the streets all over me. I was also at a stage in my life when I didn't accept the fact that I was paralyzed.

My first Caregiver was an African-American lady in her late 50s. She was excited to meet me and I'll never forget her unique raspy voice. I had no idea what to ask or what to expect. She had been doing this kind of work for some time and was engaging me on what was supposed to be going on. I was very uncomfortable for many reasons.

First of all I was allowing a total stranger into my home. Your home is supposed to be that place where you feel the most comfortable so having a stranger in my house all day was definitely different. Since she was much older than I was, a part of me looked at her as a mother figure. I've done a lot of vicious things in my life but disrespecting moms was not one of them. This made it difficult for me to feel comfortable with being myself, considering I had been used to living on my own before my paralysis.

I didn't feel comfortable asking a stranger for help. I always wondered what she thought and how she felt when she sat in my living room that day watching friend after friend, enter my bedroom and close the door. I was living in Brooklyn at the time and on my first day put most of the people that visited to work instead of her. I just felt comfortable with people who I had exchanged favors with in the past. I was afraid of rejection or her making a sarcastic remark that would trigger the rage I had hidden inside of me. I remember how awkward her sitting in my living room made my young friends and myself feel.

I didn't realize it at the time but she turned out to be one of the best Caregiver's I ever had. Unfortunately it wasn't until years later. I say she was one of my best because a couple days later I went on a verbal rampage and through her out. Fortunately my family talked the Health Care Agency into convincing her to return and she ended up caring for me for close to four years. I would get into the details about the things I put her through, but that's a whole another book.

My experience with her is what helped me to recognize the qualities of a good Caregiver. Throughout my life most of the good ones possessed the same qualities as my first. Nowadays I still have a form of anxiety when meeting a new one but it's not as bad as my first time. Now I know what to ask and what to look for.

The following are a couple of simple but very important fact-finding questions that a Client or family member should ask new Caregiver's.

1) How long have you been doing this work?

This gives a Client a really good idea of a person's experience in the field. It can get real interesting for a Client to work with a Caregiver with less than one year of experience. Taking care of a quadriplegic is a demanding job. It can also be emotionally challenging and if you do not know what to expect as a Client it could affect the longevity.

On the other hand a lack of experience could be a good thing if within the first week you believe that the Caregiver is trainable. This could create a long-lasting relationship if he/she is not lazy, loves helping people and has a great deal of patience.

2) How long have you been working with this agency?

This is a good question because it helps to determine a person's endurance. It can tell a lot about a person's job stability. A lot of Caregiver's I have encountered throughout the years do have a lot going on in their personal lives. A person with too many personal problems will have trouble maintaining a job or keeping a Client.

I also ran into quite a few who had their priorities ass backwards. For example, hanging out at a club all night knowing that you have to get up and go to work in the morning, even worse taking off from work just to go to the club. (SMH) I've found the previous example to be more common with much younger Caregiver's.

3) Have you ever worked with a quadriplegic?

Experience really matters and although every quadriplegic or Client is different there are some similarities. Everyone has their breaking points but someone who is experienced with working with quadriplegics is more likely to tolerate the mood swings and the demand of the job. But no matter how much experience or love a person may have for the job it will be a short relationship if the Client becomes verbally abusive.

I can't speak for those that are born with certain physical disabilities but if you've ever walked the earth like a normal person and then became paralyzed there is a great deal of anger and frustration. There is a level of confusion and depression that comes with waking up one day unable to do the things that you normally do.

It took me a long time to accept that I was paralyzed. I remember cursing out doctors, nurses and even family members. I would go from being extremely mad to feeling very depressed in a matter of seconds. It was difficult to accept that I would be dependent on someone to help with my basic needs for the rest of my life.

I believe that it takes a great deal of time for an individual that becomes physically impaired to accept. In many cases, a person never accepts that their lives have changed. They harbor this bitterness which shows its ugly face to the person closest to them, that being a Caregiver. Now I haven't given up on ever walking again but until then I had to learn how to live again, but differently.

You can learn a great deal about a person during the first meeting by asking the previous three questions. Then take at least 20 min., only after asking, "If it's okay to ask some personal questions," to get personal. It's good to know if a person is married, has kids and how they feel about family? And it doesn't hurt to ask what kind of music they enjoy and the things that they do on their off time.

These questions can help to find some common grounds to make the situation as comfortable as possible for the Client and Caregiver. Remember this is a stranger and as much information as a Client could get during the first meeting the more comfortable they will be. A Client should feel absolutely comfortable with the new Caregiver in order to wake up the next day and want to work with them again.

This is also a good time for a Client to share a little about them to the Caregiver. The Client should share their expectations and habits both good and bad. The Client needs the assistance so the sooner they get to know one another the better things are. A Client and Caregiver can always find something in common within the first 20 min. The more they have in common the longer the relationship could last.

Now as the Client you have to be honest with yourself and the Caregiver during this conversation even though the Caregiver might tell you some little white lies. Keep in mind this is similar to a job interview so I have found that sometimes they give answers they think might appease me. If he/she doesn't return the next day it saves both the Client and Caregiver some unnecessary headache.

It's kind of like meeting a man or woman that you're interested in for the first time. It's that initial conversation of fact-finding that makes the two people comfortable with one another. And most people

can tell after their first date if
they're going to answer the phone
on the next day.

Chapter 6

Communication

Being able to articulate your thoughts verbally is helpful in life in general. As a quadriplegic I've had a much better experience in dealing with my Caregiver's since I've matured and graduated from College. Sometimes in life the things that we are thinking doesn't come out correctly. Most of the time, we speak without thinking or say things that can be open to more than one interpretation.

In my youthful days I was very sarcastic, didn't hold my tongue back and if provoked could unleash a verbal assault on anyone including a Caregiver. I was only 20 when I had my accident and a kid from the streets so my attitude toward people in life, were much different. I've grown to know that there is a place and a time for everything. Now when I'm talking to a friend of mines that I grew up with my language is completely different than when I'm dealing with my Caregiver's.

I know this is my home but it doubles as a workplace and just like other workplace's I have to be conscious of the things that I say out loud. Most of us turn this off and on depending on where we are but some individuals can't control what comes out their mouth.

For example, I had a good friend that was a quadriplegic and didn't know how to articulate their needs very well. He always had trouble expressing his thoughts properly so when he spoke he used a great deal of profanity. It's just the way he expressed himself to everyone but something that a person could take personal. Most Caregiver's try not to take the way a Client expresses their thoughts to personal but the majority probably will.

From a Client's perspective, I believe we take Caregivers working for us for granted. Even though someone works for you doesn't mean that you have to speak to them in a disrespectful manner. Especially, when that person is someone you have to rely on to prepare meals and help with some of your most personal issues.

It's true what they say about you can catch more bees with honey than with shit (excuse my language) which leads to my next point. We don't always know which word might offend someone so before or directly after I say anything that could be perceived as offensive I simply say, "Excuse my language!" It's just a basic sign of respect that could take you a long way.

Now when I have a Caregiver that I'm on the same page with when it comes to my choice of words I do speak freely and the things that I say are not offensive. I was raised to always respect my elders so I'm conscious of my language when working with someone who's within the same range as my mother. Now that's just me. Some Clients have very little respect for their mother's therefore they probably and I'm going to say definitely will not respect anyone else. Talking reckless and foul will cause a Caregiver to never return.

The same can be said about a Caregiver in the Clients home and Lord knows I have encountered this more than a few times. I remember a time when I lived in New York and was receiving 12 hours straight of service. I was living with a young lady and usually slept a little late. The shift started at 9 AM and I didn't wake up until after 12 in the afternoon. Immediately after opening my eyes I asked the young lady I was staying with to send the Caregiver into my room.

I was just wiping the sleep out of my eyes when I asked the Caregiver who happened to be at my apartment for the first time to help me with something. It only took a couple minutes before she went back into the living room. About 10 to 15 min. later I needed something else so I called her into my bedroom again.

As she entered my room she said, "I was just in here... I hope you're not going to call me every 5 min.!" Yes, this was the sarcastic comment she made after sitting in my living room for three hours doing nothing. I was a little younger and to make a long story short within the next 5 min. she was no longer in my home.

Sarcasm can ruin the chance of a long-lasting relationship. Although most people have a little sarcasm in them it should be controlled. A Client or Caregiver may tolerate some sarcasm but everyone has their limits.

If a Client asks a Caregiver, "Can you cook?" And a Caregiver's response is "Of course I can, what do you think?!" "What do you think?!" is not necessary and sarcastic. Just because you're a woman with kids doesn't mean you know how to cook. There is a difference between being able to make a meal and knowing how to cook something tasteful.

A person that knows how to cook can make a simple dish like scrambled eggs taste scrumptious. Preparing a meal takes a great deal of communication between a Client and their Caregiver. A Caregiver should not assume that a Client likes a particular dish the same way they do. Not to mention there are probably plenty of Clients on special diets.

If a Client asks a Caregiver to help with something or can you do a particular task just answer the question. The answer should be either yes or no, but I'm willing to try if you can talk me through it. The extra sarcasm is something a Caregiver should keep for their friends, family and spouse.

As a Caregiver you're dealing with people that wake up every day having to deal with the emotional stress of a disability on top of everyday life. You should talk to your Client in a respectable manner at all times or say nothing at all. A sarcastic Client and a sarcastic Caregiver will probably not last long.

A person with a severe disability like a quadriplegic needs constant assistance. Speaking politely to a Caregiver and being thankful allows a Client to accomplish a lot more. When a Client is communicating their needs to a Caregiver it's good to be as specific as possible. The more detailed the instructions the less confusion between the two about the task at hand.

Whenever a Caregiver or Client begins to assume that the other knows something is the beginning of a misunderstanding. It's good to be clear on the task that you're asking to perform but it is as equally important for a Caregiver to be clear on what is being asked. A Caregiver can never ask too many questions so whenever there is some uncertainty about the task at hand, just ask! No question is ever too small or foolish. It's only foolish not to ask.

I would like to use cooking again in my next scenario. I once asked a Caregiver that was of Caribbean descent to cook some French toast. Instead of saying that they didn't know how to make them, this person attempted to cook what they thought was French toast. By the time it reached me, I had trouble identifying what it was.

Now I never asked if they knew how to prepare French toast and I didn't think to describe how it is made. Today I get a funny look from those that can cook when I ask, "Do you know how to make French toast?" I must also ask what ingredients they use to be sure. Sounds crazy but it beats having someone show up with some bread that they fried after dipping it in just an egg.

Seriously, a lack of knowledge does not make you stupid it makes you unaware. Even if someone knows how to make French toast as individuals talking about the ingredients can be crucial if a person has allergies or just prefer it to be prepared a specific way.

As people we take for granted that folks should know some of the basic things that we know. Unfortunately it's not always the case. When you're dealing with individuals from different backgrounds and ethnicity there will be huge differences. Everyone is raised differently and taught how to do things a particular way. To sum things up, what might be normal to one person is not normal to another.

The previous incident will continue to happen and become a problem if a Client assumes that someone knows how to prepare a meal they are used to eating. Now when the Client is unhappy with what was prepared and refuse to eat it the outcome can go many different ways.

I once had a lady slam my plate down on the table and get real belligerent before exiting my home. But the blame lies on both of us for a lack of communication. I didn't ask and the Caregiver for whatever reason didn't acknowledge that they weren't sure on how to prepare a particular meal.

Sometimes you will have to work with people of different ethnic groups. Even those with the same ethnic background can have different upbringings. It's good to always ask what a person can and cannot do especially when it comes to preparing meals.

A Caregiver should always ask a Client, "How would you like it to be prepared?" A very legitimate question since there are so many ways to prepare one particular meal. It doesn't hurt to ask what condiments a Client would prefer with a particular meal. Just because a Client had a sandwich yesterday with mayonnaise doesn't mean tomorrow they want it the same way. They might want mustard or nothing at all.

The communication should go both ways. A Client should be able to express their thoughts clearly and detailed to those helping with the task and as a Caregiver you must be bold and willing to ask.

Most of the problems I've experienced had a lot to do with a lack of communication. Most individuals with a physical disability are still pretty sharp mentally. A Caregiver should ask as many questions as necessary. It's a form of respecting a Client's ability to think and make decisions. Individuals with severe physical disabilities such as a quadriplegic need to be allowed to do what they are capable of doing. It is emotionally therapeutic for someone with a severe physical disability to be able to make their own decisions whether they are good or bad but not deadly.

I didn't always know how to communicate my thoughts respectably but worked on it over time. It is something that an individual can improve on.

Finally what most people really don't know about communication is that listening is very important. A Client should listen to the opinions and thoughts of their Caregiver's. Even though a Client may not agree with everything they say sometimes they come up with some very good suggestions. Some of the Caregiver's ideas could makes life easier. No matter what the age gap is between a Client and Caregiver you both can learn something from one another. And no matter what the level of education we can all learn how to express our thoughts to someone in a respectable and productive manner.

Chapter 7

The Client (Quadriplegic)

There are many different types of Clients that receive service from a Caregiver. I can only write about my experiences and give my opinions from the perspective of a quadriplegic. But on behalf of all Clients we "need" the assistance so if you don't have any patience or compassion, becoming a Caregiver might not be something for you.

As a quadriplegic I've struggled with depression. Emotionally I'm doing well but I still have times throughout the year when being paralyzed coupled with everyday life sneaks up on me. I can become moody and extremely sensitive to everything that's going on in my life. It is a time when my tolerance for sarcasm and foolishness is low.

When a Caregiver has been around me for some time they can tell when I'm having a bad day. It's also something that I let them know when they arrive at my home for work. I need them to understand that anything I say or do, should not be taken personal. Sometimes my frustration over being disabled gets the best of me and I usually say very little. These are times when I count on my Caregiver for compassion and emotional support.

Life is difficult for individuals that don't have spinal cord injuries so imagine the difficulty a quadriplegic has on a daily basis. It can get rough having to deal with everyday life on top of having a physical disability. Although I am a quadriplegic most of my emotions are not related to my paralysis.

At the end of the day I am still a human being with all of my naturally emotions. If someone says something to me that I don't like it makes me angry, if someone breaks something in my home it bothers me and when death hits close to home my heart aches. These are things that when combined with my paralysis could trigger my bad side.

As I've gotten older and closer to God, I am more appreciative of life and therefore when I have emotions of anger or disappointment I pray on it before letting it go. Every day is a gift from God and I do my best not to spend it complaining about my new lifestyle and all that comes with it. I stay positive because no one really likes to be around a dark cloud.

Nevertheless most of my disgruntled emotions are caused by normal everyday life and not my paralysis. I say this because I believe that most Caregiver's think that people that are paralyzed are bitter. This might be the case for many but not all.

Just like everyone grieves differently, every Client especially quadriplegics deal with their paralysis differently. There are two types of quadriplegics, those that are either active quads or non-active. The non-active quads have a difficult time accepting their paralysis and are usually extremely depressed which leads to a lack of social activities. They're usually bitter about their paralysis and take out their frustrations on those closest to them.

When I first became paralyzed I spent 20 months in the hospital. I spent over 12 months in a rehabilitation center around hundreds of people with physical and mental disabilities. When I finally got discharged to my own apartment I was a little scared. It was time for me to get back to being sociable and living my life. I was afraid to go places that my wheelchair might not be able to get in to. I didn't want to feel embarrassed and a part of me wasn't happy with how I looked as a person in a wheelchair.

I was comfortable in the hospital around people like me but returning back to society was completely different. I found excuses and lost interest in doing things that I normally did before becoming paralyzed. I remember staying in my home for months at a time, especially during the winter.

When I first came out of the hospital in 1991, I moved to Georgia and they didn't even have Health Care Agencies or Caregiver's. I relied on a lady friend and my family for my first year out of the hospital. I wasn't that active at all because once my family helped with my personal needs I didn't want to burden them with helping me with any extra activities.

After feeling like a burden on my girlfriend and family I moved back to New York where they had more Health Care Agencies and Caregiver's to help me live independently. My Caregivers, family and friends tried desperately to encourage me to go places. A Caregiver that's in it for the money might like a Client that is not active because they are in a normal routine most of the time unlike an active quadriplegic. An active quadriplegic routine changes constantly depending on their goals and ambitions in life.

It took me some time but now I am what most people consider an active quad. This is someone who after their paralysis decided to accept it and move on with life as normal as possible. My routine constantly changes because I'm always looking for something to get into. It took me almost 2 years after my diagnosis to really accept my condition and get back to living.

Since I've accepted my paralysis my life has changed drastically. I pretty much do everything that I would have if I could walk. I've even done some things since I've been paralyzed that I didn't do when I was walking. For example I've flown on an airplane several times since being paralyzed without anyone escorting me. I had never been on a plane before in my life but the experience was an interesting adventure.

From the time I entered the airport in New York and until I landed in Georgia the airline accommodations were wonderful. The airline's staff helped me on the airplane first, before helping to transfer me from my wheelchair to an actual seat. Once in the air one of the stewardess helped with drinks and food while checking on me constantly to make sure I was comfortable. There were times when I got on a plane with very few passengers and was allowed to ride first class which was much more comfortable than coach.

Up until I was about 30 I attended several premier clubs throughout New York City with the assistance of my friends and family. They are truly the backbone to my movements. Everyone who has a physical disability, especially a quadriplegic, needs a supporting team. It's my supporting team that keeps me wanting to enjoy life. Although my family and friends keep me enjoying life my Caregiver's contribute greatly.

Since I've been paralyzed I went back to school where I received a couple of College degrees. Attending College is difficult for individuals without disabilities so it was even harder being a quadriplegic. Going to school was difficult at first. God eventually blessed me with a good Caregiver. I had an excellent one for 5 of my 6 1/2 years spent in school. I would not have been able to accomplish that task without the assistance of a stable Caregiver.

This person was patient and extremely compassionate to my situation. Before this Caregiver I had a couple that didn't like getting me dress and escorting me to school, especially when I had to travel across the city on public buses. Getting up and out the house to attend school was emotionally therapeutic. It kept my mind off of being paralyzed and I was no longer ashamed of being in public.

Every now and then I would run into someone who'd asked me did I go to a regular school. It doesn't offend me because they don't know but the answer is always yes. I was enrolled in Medgar Evers College, a city University located in New York and it was and still is a school for anyone. I was the only one in all my classes that was actually in a wheelchair. I was always positioned in the front of the class and the professors in the school were accommodating to my needs. They also had the same expectations for me as everyone else.

I met some wonderful people and learned a great deal about myself and life in general. It's also where I got introduced to some software called Dragon NaturallySpeaking that allows me to use a computer independently. I think God every day for the technology and the time that were living in. There was a time when someone with a severe spinal cord injury like me was unable to live life independently let alone enjoy the things they did before their paralysis.

I've been on a ski trip even though I was unable to ski. Today there is adaptive equipment for people with disabilities to enjoy the slopes. I was in a relationship and thought that it was something nice for my lady friend. Just because I have a disability, doesn't mean that she should be deprived of activities requiring mobility.

Some might ask, what did I get out of the trip? Well I enjoyed being up in the mountains with my lady friend, surrounded by snow, drinking hot chocolate and chopping it up with my friends. And yes I did say I took a lady friend of mines on a ski trip. (Smile)

Ever since the founding of the ADA (Americans with Disabilities Act) in the early 1990s, life for individuals with disabilities and especially severe spinal cord injuries has improved. Not to get technical, it's basically a law that makes it illegal to have a public establishment that doesn't accommodate individuals with disabilities. All new buildings being constructed must be wheelchair accessible and disability friendly. Most of the places I go like the movies and grocery stores are wheelchair accessible. New York City has installed elevators at several major train stations and added a wheel chair lift on every city bus, both I've experienced.

Everywhere I go people are extremely generous and accommodating. One of my most recent and exciting adventures was a trip I took to Florida. I was in Tampa at a family reunion that was taking place on the beach.

To my surprise the beach had a special chair designed for people that are paralyzed that rolled across the sand. With the assistance of my family I was able to get my feet wet in the ocean. It was a big deal for me because I thought that I would never be able to put my feet in ocean water again. I've been to several beaches since becoming paralyzed but never across the sand.

Just because I have a physical disability doesn't mean I have mental challenges. I'm able to conduct a productive life with the assistance of a Caregiver. But it must be a person with a great deal of patience and love for the job especially when working with an active quad. Being an active quad is not just about going places but it also means being active around my home.

Now I've only touched on a few things that both a Caregiver and Client can do to have a long lasting relationship. I do believe out of everything I mentioned that there are two very important tips.

First of all, good communication can cut down on some unnecessary confrontation. Both the Caregiver and Client should constantly ask one another questions. Being able to communicate well is something everyone can learn.

Secondly, the Client should not be unwilling to make some minor adjustments. The Client's home is also a workplace so making a few minor adjustments to make the Caregiver comfortable is always a plus. The more comfortable the

Caregiver is with the Client the more productive they will be.

While writing this someone stated that my title sounded like a Client was in a relationship with the Caregiver. My response was "it is a relationship". It's a working relationship that could turn into a friendship if the two individuals have a lot in common. And just like any other relationship, you get out of it... what you put in! As a Client, it doesn't hurt to be kind, considerate and appreciative of the services. A simple "thank you" from time to time can take a Client and Caregiver relationship a long way.

Even though Caregiver's help individuals with physical disabilities to live an independent life it's the family and friends that helps a Client enjoy life. We are all people who go through different emotions. As an active quad I am too busy thinking of my next move to be bitter about my paralysis. Staying busy keeps my mind off of being paralyzed and becoming a bitter person. There are characteristics about ourselves that we cannot change. I think Clients and Caregiver's need to be more understanding toward one another's personal situations.

The Caregiver's job is to come to a person's home and assist the Client with everyday living. I believe a Client's job is to be courteous and respectful to the people that are helping them, live life!

There is no perfect Caregiver or Client but you could always find one whose flaws don't outweigh the benefits. It's been over 20 years since I've been paralyzed and I can honestly say that having a stable Caregiver is important to any Client, especially a quadriplegic.

In conclusion, a Caregiver and a Client can have a long, healthy working relationship. It can be demanding and challenging for a Caregiver. Most Caregivers in the profession cannot handle the demand just like most quadriplegic will never accept their new lifestyle.